ALEXANDER ROBINSON ELEMENTARY
11849 - 238B Street
Maple Ridge, B C V4R 2T8
Ph: 604-463-3035 Fax: 604-463-0667

Managing **Anxiety**

Hal Marcovitz

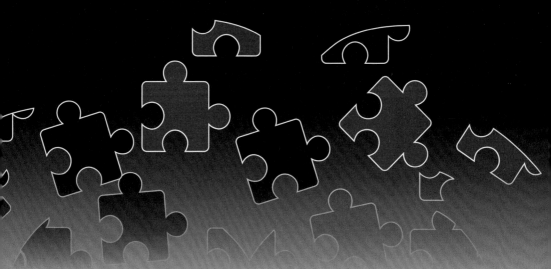

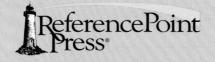

ReferencePoint
Press®

San Diego, CA

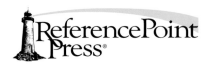

© 2022 ReferencePoint Press, Inc.
Printed in the United States

For more information, contact:
ReferencePoint Press, Inc.
PO Box 27779
San Diego, CA 92198
www.ReferencePointPress.com

LIBRARY OF CONGRESS CATALOGING-IN-PUBLICATION DATA

Names: Marcovitz, Hal, author
 Title: Managing anxiety / by Hal Marcovitz.
Description: San Diego, CA : ReferencePoint Press, Inc., 2022. | Series: Managing mental health Includes bibliographical references and index.
Identifiers: LCCN 2021013121 (print) | LCCN 2021013122 (ebook) | ISBN 9781678201067 (library binding) | ISBN 9781678201074 (ebook)
Subjects: LCSH: Anxiety disorders--Juvenile literature. | Anxiety disorders--Treatment--Juvenile literature.
Classification: LCC RC531 .M337 2022 (print) | LCC RC531 (ebook) | DDC 616.85/22--dc23
LC record available at https://lccn.loc.gov/2021013121
LC ebook record available at https://lccn.loc.gov/2021013122

Contents

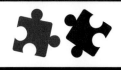

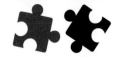

Even Superheroes Suffer from Anxiety

Actor Ryan Reynolds burst into stardom in 2016 when he portrayed the title character in the film *Deadpool*—the story of a quirky, wisecracking superhero. The movie proved to be enormously popular, garnering more than $780 million at the box office. The film spawned a 2018 sequel, *Deadpool 2*. A third film in the series, *Deadpool 3*, is tentatively planned for release in 2023. According to *Rolling Stone* magazine film critic Peter Travers, "*Deadpool* is party time for action junkies and Reynolds may just have found the role that makes his career."[1]

But although Reynolds's character on the screen delights audiences and impresses critics, the actor portraying the role of the screwball yet heroic Deadpool is a much different person. Reynolds suffers from severe bouts of anxiety. Prior to being interviewed by reporters or appearing as a guest on television talk shows, Reynolds endures extreme nausea and often must vomit. At times, he is so nervous that he cannot eat. The intense hype that the movie studio orchestrated in the months prior to the release of *Deadpool* only added to his anxiety. After learning the studio planned to spend millions of dollars promoting the film as a blockbuster, Reynolds admitted to being terrified it would fail at the box office. Reynolds says, "When there's built-in expectation your brain always processes that as danger."[2]

Anxiety affects millions of people worldwide. Typically, people experience moments of anxiety when they are confronted by issues or problems that cause them to fear they will in some way fail. In many cases, anxiety can be a more constant and even daily affliction. In such cases, these feelings of fear can be classified as anxiety disorders that may require professional counseling and even prescription medications. People who suffer from anxiety disorders may find themselves so overcome with fear that they experience physical effects, such as a racing heartbeat, intense perspiration, an inability to sleep, and, as in Reynolds's case, nausea and vomiting.

Meditation Helps Reduce Anxiety

Anxiety is a condition that Reynolds has endured for much of his life. Growing up in Vancouver, British Columbia, Reynolds described his home life as an often-volatile atmosphere due to a father who always seemed angry. Drawn to acting, Reynolds traveled to Hollywood after dropping out of college in his freshman year and soon landed a role in the short-lived television sitcom *Two Guys, a Girl and a Pizza Place*. It was during the production of the show that Reynolds first noticed his fears taking over his life. He often woke from sleep in the middle of the night, frozen with fear that he would flounder on set or that his acting career would end in failure. To deal with his fears, Reynolds turned to drugs. "I was partying and just trying to make myself vanish in some way,"[3] he says. But after a friend died of a drug overdose, Reynolds gave up drugs and looked for other ways to deal with his anxiety.

"When there's built-in expectation your brain always processes that as danger."[2]

—Ryan Reynolds, actor

Of course, his career did not derail. Reynolds acted in many roles prior to the release of *Deadpool*, and in the years since the release of the original film, he has made many other successful films. But his anxiety has persisted. It was during the production of the original *Deadpool* film that Reynolds feared for his health due to his constant symptoms of nausea and vomiting and sought a diagnosis for his ills. A doctor soon detected that Reynolds did not suffer from a physical ailment but, rather, was afflicted with an anxiety disorder. To deal with the fears that torture him, he has tried meditation. People who meditate attempt to focus their minds on specific objects or positive ideas as a way to eliminate the jumbled thoughts that terrify them and cause anxiety. Scientific studies have shown that meditation can help reduce anxiety. "Our results show a clear reduction in anxiety in the first hour after the meditation session, and our preliminary results suggest that anxiety was significantly lower one week after the meditation session,"[4] says biologist John J. Durocher, who headed a 2018 study into meditation therapy at Michigan Technological University in Houghton.

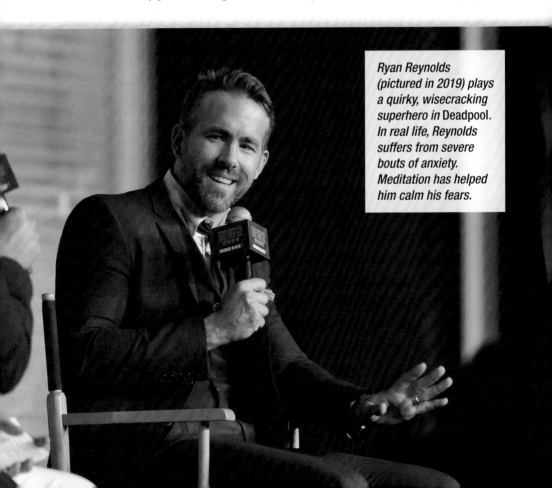

Ryan Reynolds (pictured in 2019) plays a quirky, wisecracking superhero in Deadpool. *In real life, Reynolds suffers from severe bouts of anxiety. Meditation has helped him calm his fears.*

Hiding Behind His Characters

When Reynolds practices meditation, he often relies on a phone app that helps guide users through their sessions. It also offers specific steps to help quell their fears in connection with health, relationships, and job performance. Reynolds also finds it helpful that when he sits down for interviews or meets other people who may prompt his fears to surface, he falls into character. He is able to hide behind a role he has played on-screen. "I turn on this knucklehead, and he kind of takes over," he says. "That's [a] great self-defense mechanism."[5]

"Our preliminary results suggest that anxiety was significantly lower one week after the meditation session."[4]

—John J. Durocher, biologist

Although this particular strategy is not available to most people, Reynolds's experience illustrates how widespread anxiety and anxiety disorders can be. They afflict even very successful Hollywood actors. And although anxiety remains a very real part of Reynolds's life, and the lives of millions of others, it can be a manageable condition—with hard work and, when needed, professional guidance.

Chapter One

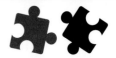

What Is Everyday Anxiety?

Whenever advertising copywriter Scott Muska meets a woman at a party or similar social occasion and decides he would like to ask her out on a date, he always takes the first step by sending her a text later that day or evening. He admits, though, that when he asks someone out on a date through a text, he finds himself filled with anxiety. "You get super panicky in the time between your sending of an important text message to a romantic interest and . . . [her] response," he says. "While you're waiting with bated breath, a slew of super-negative thoughts race through your head about why she hasn't answered yet and about what terrible response you might receive. . . . Does she hate me now? Did I come on too strong?"[6]

A generation ago, when few people carried mobile phones and texting was not common, Muska would likely have had to ask for a date face-to-face, often within a few minutes of meeting someone to whom he felt attracted. And if she turned him down, the drama would have been over quickly, and very likely, Muska would have been able to shrug off the experience and move on with his life. But in today's world, when so many people are connected to their phones and texting is a big part of virtually everyone's life, Muska has found a way to make himself anxious and fretful over the simple act of asking a young woman for a date.

Muska is not alone. So-called texting anxiety has become a common part of life. With texting, a vacuum of uncertainty exists between the moment the text is sent and the moment a reply is received. Whether that vacuum of uncertainty lasts for a few seconds, a few minutes, a few hours, or a few days, the texter is likely to feel somewhat anxious or worried about whether the answer will be the one he or she hopes for. Psychologist Lucie Hemmen describes this common response:

> Let's say you were texting with a crush who suddenly drops off in the conversation. You text a question mark and wait . . . but nothing. You then wonder if you said something offensive so you re-read the text string searching for clues. You think you identified a problem, a comment you made that could have come off wrong. Now your thoughts (mental distress) stimulate a flood of worry (more mental distress), which causes your stomach to sink and your chest to tighten (physical distress). You feel irritable, nervous, scared, embarrassed (emotional distress), and you snap hard on your little sister when she comes into your room to ask an innocent question (behavioral distress). This is the head-to-toe work of anxiety in action.[7]

Anxiety Can Be Good

Texting anxiety is an example of "everyday anxiety"—a form of anxiety that is a routine part of life for many people. There are many reasons people lapse into moments of anxiety. Awaiting a text response is just one of these. Other reasons for anxious feelings include concerns about paying bills or landing a job. Some people feel anxious in social situations, such as parties, school dances, or even sitting with friends around the table in the cafeteria. They are worried they will say or do something that will cause themselves to be embarrassed in front of others. Health issues can contribute to people's feelings of anxiety. Parents who worry about the health and well-being of their children can become consumed by anxiety. Even being late for an appointment can trigger an episode of anxiety. Young people can feel anxiety when they go out on a date with someone new. Others who may have to make an important presentation at a business meeting can suffer from anxiety as the date of the meeting approaches. Performers can feel anxious as they prepare to walk onstage, particularly on opening night. Finally, people can find themselves caught up in anxiety as they walk into an unfamiliar situation.

Virtually everybody feels anxious moments from time to time. In fact, minor feelings of anxiety can be beneficial. According to Zee Krstic, the health editor for *Good Housekeeping* magazine, "We all sometimes feel anxiety—a sense of unease or worry

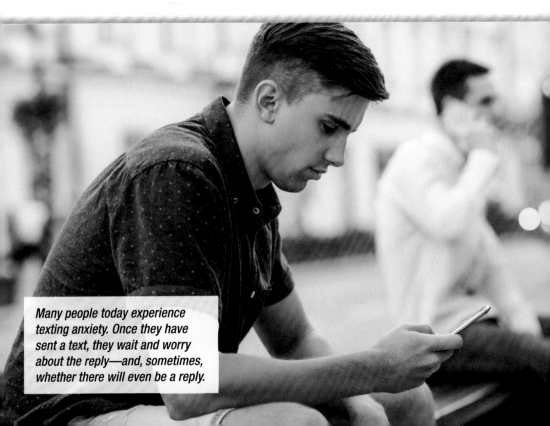

Many people today experience texting anxiety. Once they have sent a text, they wait and worry about the reply—and, sometimes, whether there will even be a reply.

about something uncertain in the future—which is a good thing: A bit of performance anxiety, for example, which can manifest as apprehension or even dread, might motivate you to hunker down and prepare for a test or a speech."[8] In fact, people who are too at ease with difficult situations might not be fully considering the seriousness of their problems or challenges. Thus, their aloof attitudes could cause them to miss deadlines, turn in substandard work, or even forget their assignments are due. And so, as Krstic says, a little anxiety can actually work in people's favor.

> "A bit of performance anxiety, for example, which can manifest as apprehension or even dread, might motivate you to hunker down and prepare for a test or a speech."[8]
>
> —Zee Krstic, health editor for *Good Housekeeping* magazine

Fight or Flight

Everyone has uniquely personal reasons for letting feelings of fear or worry bubble to the surface. And although anxiety may be caused by these individual reasons, people are generally able to confront their fears and find ways to cope. As authors David Mellinger, a clinical social worker, and Steven Jay Lynn, a psychologist, write,

> "Normal" means of relieving and controlling anxiety often work well enough to ease nervousness, fearfulness, and tension. Many people are satisfied with the calming, heartening effects of prayer or affirmation or the rejuvenating power of healthy exercise, or else they successfully "white-knuckle" their way through anxiety-provoking events and relationships. And many people are capable of problem-solving and toning down episodes of stress and can somehow transform excessive anxiety into creativity, energy, and good works.[9]

How well people handle their own anxieties often depends on how they react to a mental and physical function known as the fight-or-flight response. When people encounter unfamiliar situations, the fight-or-flight response guides their reaction. If they find themselves willing to confront the situation, they are likely to experience the fight response. That does not necessarily mean they will ball their hands into fists and throw a punch. Rather, it means they are prepared to deal with the stress and offer rational responses to the situation they are facing. On the other hand, if they are overcome with anxiety, it is likely they will experience the flight response, meaning they will do whatever they can to avoid confronting the issue that sparked the flight response.

When people are first confronted by unfamiliar situations, their initial reactions are tripped by a component of the human brain known as the amygdala, which is a tiny almond-shaped organ that sparks a person's emotional responses. The amygdala sends a message of distress to a second component of the brain, the hypothalamus, which acts as a command center, sending signals to the rest of the body. Based on the message transmitted by the amygdala, the hypothalamus may respond by quickening a person's heartbeat, increasing blood pressure, or making the person

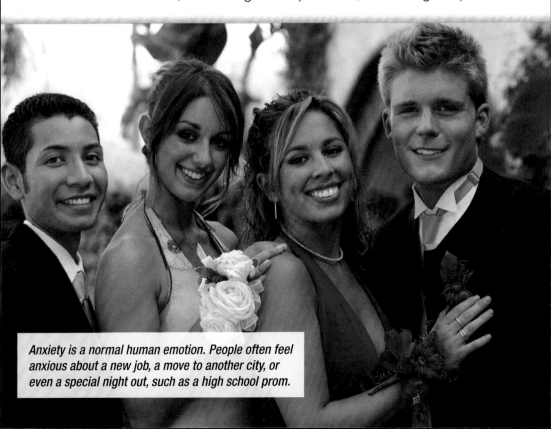

Anxiety is a normal human emotion. People often feel anxious about a new job, a move to another city, or even a special night out, such as a high school prom.

take short, quick breaths. All of these physical reactions reflect the degree of anxiety the person is experiencing.

A third component of the brain, the hippocampus, also participates in the response. The hippocampus is the storehouse for a person's long-term memories. As such, the hippocampus may serve to moderate the signals sent by the amygdala. If the person has experienced the situation before, the hippocampus will help guide his or her response. The hippocampus may, for example, remind the person that he or she had similar experiences in the past and there is no danger.

Conversely, the hippocampus might remind a person that there could be very real or imagined danger ahead. Mellinger and Lynn recall the story of a young woman named Lisa. After returning home from a Halloween party where she and others had watched a horror movie, Lisa found her anxiety growing after hearing an unusual knocking sound coming from her back door. Since the most recent memory stored in her hippocampus included images of a cinematic ax murderer stalking his victims, her fight-or-flight response kicked in the moment she heard the unusual sound. As Mellinger and Lynn explain,

> A mere instant after the knock on the door triggered her emotional response, Lisa's hippocampus provided her with relevant memories as well as the "emergency response cards" or automatic thoughts. More precisely, if she were not too jumpy, Lisa might think, "Oh, that's just my oddball neighbor," but when Lisa is truly wired, her hippocampus boosts her uneasiness with mental images of deranged prowlers breaking into her house.[10]

Anxiety in Young People

Of course, people react differently to different situations. Someone else who attended that party and saw the same film may have had a far different response to a knocking sound than Lisa experienced. In other words, an event that triggers the fight-or-flight

13

Social Media Anxiety

Social media has engaged millions of people in online forums where they share their interests, give feedback to one another, and stay connected with friends who may be separated from them by long distances. But social media can also spark anxiety among its users.

The network news program *Today* surveyed seven thousand American mothers and found that 42 percent suffered from what it referred to as "Pinterest stress": stress caused by not being creative enough to merit the admiration of others on the social media platform. Pinterest posts are devoted to recipes, sewing patterns, designs for household knickknacks, and similar creative pursuits. According to *Today*, "Symptoms include staying up until 3 a.m. clicking through photos of exquisite hand-made birthday party favors even though you'll end up buying yours at the dollar store, or sobbing quietly into a burnt mess of expensive ingredients that were supposed to be adorable bunny cookies for the school bake sale."

Moreover, a 2015 study of 1,095 Facebook users by psychologists in Denmark found that people's anxieties decrease when they stop using Facebook. "It was demonstrated that taking a break from Facebook has positive effects on the two dimensions of well-being: our life satisfaction increases and our emotions become more positive," the study found.

Quoted in Maureen O'Connor, "The Six Major Anxieties of Social Media," *The Cut* (blog), *New York*, May 14, 2013. www.thecut.com.

Morten Tromholt, "The Facebook Experiment: Quitting Facebook Leads to Higher Levels of Well-Being," *Cyberpsychology, Behavior, and Social Networking*, November 1, 2016. https://pubmed.ncbi.nlm.nih.gov.

response in one person might not do so in another person. Courtenay Hameister, who formerly hosted a nationally broadcast radio show, believes she experienced her first fight-or-flight response at the age of eight when she ventured out to the end of a diving board over a public pool. Looking down at the surface of the pool, 16 feet (5 m) below, Hameister says she suddenly felt a deep sense of anxiety about making the jump. But also, she says, the other young swimmers on the ladder behind her were growing impatient, taunting her to jump. Therefore, whereas Hameister's brain was prompting her to run away, many young people behind her were more than willing to dash off the end of the diving board.

In this case, though, Hameister's anxiety was intensified because she knew she would have to endure the stares and snickers of the other swimmers as she descended the ladder of the diving board. She realized that she could never find the courage to make the jump—to stay and put up a fight against the frightening diving board. She says, "You already know you can't do it, and now instead of working up the courage to jump, you're working up the courage to walk the gauntlet of searing side-eyes you'll endure on the Climb of Shame down to the scorching pavement. This is where you learned it: You are not the leaping type."[11]

Katie Hurley, a clinical social worker, says teens and young children often suffer from anxiety because many experiences are new to them. Essentially, they do not have a lot of prior memories stored in their brains that can provide them with experiences on which to rely for direction. She says they may be going out on dates for the first time, speaking in public, or playing in important games for their high school or middle school teams. Or, as Hameister's experience illustrates, they may have ventured out to the end of a diving board for the first time in their lives.

Because they have not had a lot of experience in dealing with stressful situations, they can easily be troubled by the fear of the unknown. "All teens experience some amount of anxiety at times," says Hurley.

> Anxiety is actually a normal reaction to stress, and sometimes it helps teens deal with tense or overwhelming situations. For many teens, things like public speaking, final exams, important athletic competitions, or even going out on a date can cause feelings of apprehension and uneasiness. They may also experience an increase in heartbeat or excessive sweating. That's how the brain responds to anxious feelings.[12]

Girls and Anxiety

Although feelings of anxiety can confront all young people, research by mental health experts shows that girls may suffer more than boys. Psychologist Lisa Damour says girls may suffer

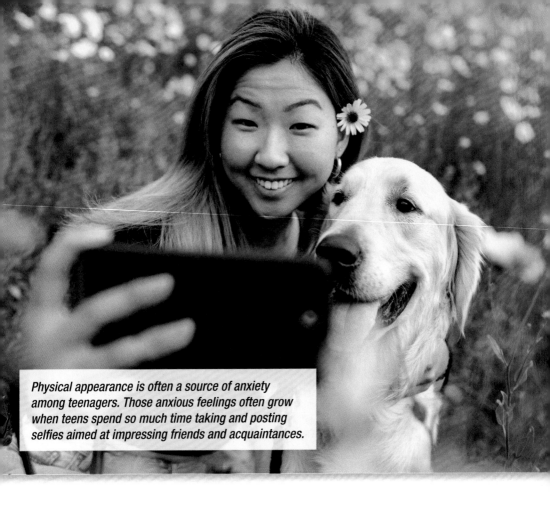

Physical appearance is often a source of anxiety among teenagers. Those anxious feelings often grow when teens spend so much time taking and posting selfies aimed at impressing friends and acquaintances.

more from anxiety because they tend to brood over their problems longer and deeper than what is commonly found among boys. According to Damour,

> Studies show . . . that girls are more likely than boys to worry about how they are doing in school. While it's nothing new for our daughters to strive to live up to the expectations of adults, I now hear regularly about girls who are so fearful of disappointing their teachers that they skip sleep to do extra-credit work for points they don't need. Research also tells us that our daughters, more than our sons, worry about how they look. Though teens have always experienced moments of high anxiety about their physical appearance, we are raising the first generation

that can, and often does, devote hours at a time to fretfully curating and posting selfies in the hopes that they will receive an avalanche of likes.[13]

What is also common—among teens of both sexes—is not knowing what to do about their feelings of anxiety. In these situations, a common response is to run away or avoid whatever is creating the anxiety.

Running away from an uncomfortable or unfamiliar situation could include making bad decisions. Damour, who serves as the school psychologist at a high school in Shaker Heights, Ohio, cites the case of one student, a sixteen-year-old girl named Dana. Dana, Damour explains, went to a party but soon found herself unnerved by the other young people there. She felt many of the other partygoers were sketchy. She reacted to her anxiety by drinking beer and shots of hard liquor—so much, in fact, that she passed out and had to be taken to an emergency room. This was her way of avoiding the uncomfortable situation. "It wasn't a good scene," Dana told Damour. "But I knew my friends wanted to stay, so I didn't know what to do. Obviously, I shouldn't have done what I did."[14]

As Dana's experience illustrates, anxiety is a part of the lives of many people. Some anxiety is self-inflicted. Scott Muska has fallen into the habit of asking for dates by sending texts. And as he waits for an answer, he finds himself troubled by his fears of rejection.

> "We are raising the first generation that can, and often does, devote hours at a time to fretfully curating and posting selfies in the hopes that they will receive an avalanche of likes."[13]
>
> —Lisa Damour, psychologist

Lisa's anxiety was also self-inflicted. Had she not watched that horror movie earlier in the evening, she likely would have shrugged off that knocking sound at her back door. Instead, she immediately conjured up the anxious thought that she was being stalked by a killer. Courtenay Hameister's moment of anxiety illustrates

Anxiety and Climate Change

Climate change—the warming of earth's atmosphere due to pollution from carbon-based fuels such as oil, natural gas, and coal—has prompted widespread anxiety among people who fear for their futures. Scientists say climate change is contributing to more and deadlier storms, hastening species decline, and threatening coastal cities due to rising sea levels. A 2020 poll by the American Psychiatric Association found that a majority of Americans are somewhat or extremely anxious about their futures due to the impacts of climate change.

Young people are particularly anxious about the effects of climate change. The study found that 67 percent of people between the ages of eighteen and twenty-three and 63 percent of people between the ages of twenty-four and thirty-nine are somewhat or very concerned about climate change. Older people are less concerned: 58 percent of people between the ages of forty and fifty-five and 42 percent of people who are older than fifty-six are either somewhat or very concerned about climate change.

British psychotherapist Caroline Hickman found positive news in the study. Hickman suggested that a growing anxiety over climate change may prompt political leaders to take definitive action to curb carbon pollution. "I'd kind of wonder why somebody wasn't feeling anxious," she says.

Quoted in Christine Ro, "The Harm from Worrying About Climate Change," *The Future* (blog), BBC, October 10, 2019. www.bbc.com.

how the fight-or-flight response can be sparked by the seemingly harmless act of walking out to the end of a diving board at a public pool. And in Dana's case, her moment of anxiety led her to make a bad decision—drinking alcohol at a party because she felt uncomfortable in the company of strangers. Anxiety is a condition that can affect anyone who is exposed to a stressful situation. And although a little bit of anxiety can help many people perform better, for others, anxiety can have very undesirable consequences.

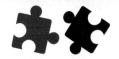

Chapter Two

What Happens When Anxiety Becomes a Disorder?

When Gina was a young girl, she had few friends. Gina recalled that her mother often explained away her lack of friends by saying, "She's just a little shy."[15] At school, Gina did not like participating in class. She never raised her hand when the teacher asked for an answer from the class. When called on by the teacher, Gina often froze up in fear. At lunchtime, Gina always ate by herself. She frequently suffered from stomachaches and often begged her parents to let her stay home from school.

Even as she grew older, Gina found herself spending much of her time alone. She never dated. After finding a job as a pharmacy technician, she always declined invitations from coworkers to join them for lunch, making excuses for why she preferred to eat alone. At one point, after declining an invitation to eat lunch with her coworkers, she overheard one of them say, "Gina thinks she's too good for us."[16] That comment sent Gina to the restroom, where she collapsed in tears.

Gina does not think of herself as better than other people. Rather, she suffers from anxiety. Her anxiety is so extreme that it can be classified as a mental illness known as social anxiety disorder. More than simple shyness, social anxiety disorder causes people to feel intense fear when they are forced into situations in which they have to interact with others. Social anxiety disorder is characterized by irrational fears of being humiliated. During conversations with others, people who suffer from social anxiety disorder may fear making inappropriate comments and being scorned or simply not knowing what to say and remaining silent in response to a question. As a result, they may avoid taking part in conversations, contributing to class discussions, or offering their ideas in groups.

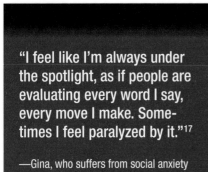

"I feel like I'm always under the spotlight, as if people are evaluating every word I say, every move I make. Sometimes I feel paralyzed by it."[17]

—Gina, who suffers from social anxiety disorder

And, if forced into such situations, they may respond by succumbing to a condition known as a panic attack—as Gina did when she ran to the restroom at work. Gina says, "I feel like I'm always under the spotlight, as if people are evaluating every word I say, every move I make. Sometimes I feel paralyzed by it. I just know I'm going to do or say something to make others disapprove of me. I don't want to go on like this."[17]

When Anxiety Affects Mental Health

The level of anxiety suffered by Gina is much more intense than the anxiety most people experience. It is not uncommon, for instance, for a person learning to drive to feel anxious. After all, new drivers must learn many skills as they take the wheel, such as how the accelerator and brakes work, when to engage the turn signals and headlights, how to turn on the windshield wipers, and so on. Moreover, there is also a level of fear and uncertainty as they venture out into traffic for the first time. But as they grow more familiar with the controls and become more comfortable operating their vehicles in city traffic, eventually their fears ease.

But for many people, the anxiety never passes. Anxiety becomes a regular and even daily part of their lives. The periods of anxiety they endure are longer than those brief moments when people find themselves under normal levels of stress. The intensity of those episodes is much more powerful than a typical episode of anxiety that a new driver may experience.

Moreover, the symptoms of anxiety are more extreme for someone with an anxiety disorder. Whereas people who find themselves in anxious moments may break out in a sweat or notice their hearts beating faster, the physical symptoms that afflict sufferers of anxiety disorders are often much more intense. Sufferers of anxiety disorders may find themselves trembling. They may need to vomit. They may be overcome with a feeling of weariness. Many sufferers of anxiety disorder endure long nights of insomnia. The mental and emotional stress of these feelings can lead to a sort of paralysis or inability to function. According to the American Addiction Centers, an organization based in San Diego, California,

Anxiety is considered normal and adaptive when it serves to improve peoples' functioning or well-being. In contrast,

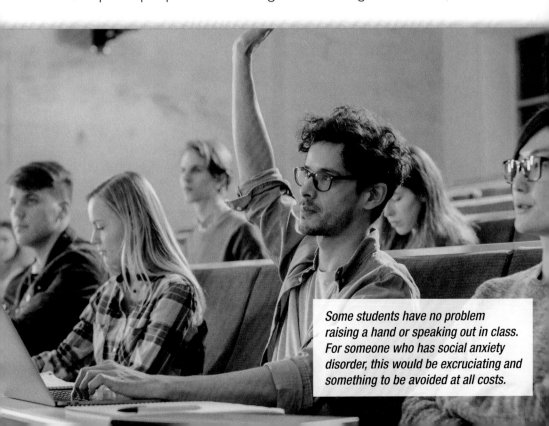

Some students have no problem raising a hand or speaking out in class. For someone who has social anxiety disorder, this would be excruciating and something to be avoided at all costs.

abnormal anxiety is a chronic condition that impairs people's functioning and interferes with their well-being. This impairment causes them significant distress. There are specific symptoms that accompany each anxiety disorder. However, the main criteria used to distinguish normal anxiety from an anxiety disorder is that it results in significant distress, or impairs social, occupational, or other important areas of functioning.[18]

As Cheryl Carmin, a psychologist at Ohio State University, explains, "What makes this a diagnosable condition is that it causes a person to be distressed, or the anxiety interferes with a person's life. Most people are anxious before a job interview, but for the person who has an anxiety disorder, they may cancel the interview altogether due to their fear about what the interviewer may think about them."[19]

Obsessive Compulsive Disorder

Many psychologists regard obsessive compulsive disorder (OCD) as an anxiety disorder. People afflicted with OCD experience constant and distressing thoughts (obsessions) that cause them to repeatedly act out behaviors (compulsions). One common form of OCD involves an obsession with cleanliness. This obsession turns into compulsive, or repeated, smoothing out of wrinkles in slipcovers, wiping dust off of shelves, sweeping of floors, and so on. According to the National Institute of Mental Health, OCD affects one in forty adults and one in one hundred children in America.

Psychologist Graham C.L. Davey says people who suffer from OCD often harbor a deep sense of guilt, believing that if they do not take precautions something bad will happen to others. He says, "Checking the stove is off prevents a potential gas explosion, checking the doors and windows are locked prevents the house from being burgled, washing one's hands until they are raw prevents contamination and the possible spread of diseases to others…Not only do individuals with OCD tend to feel responsible for ensuring that bad things don't happen, but they also have a highly inflated sense of responsibility that evokes guilt and shame at the possibility of bad things happening if their compulsive rituals are not completed properly and thoroughly."

Graham C.L. Davey, "The Psychology of OCD," *Psychology Today*, December 3, 2019. www.psychologytoday.com.

More than One Type of Disorder

There is more than one type of anxiety disorder. Although these disorders each have their own unique set of characteristics, they all involve extreme levels of anxiety and interfere in some fashion with the person's ability to pursue a normal life. Gina has social anxiety disorder, a condition that was first identified in 1980 when psychologists classified the various forms of anxiety disorders. According to the Anxiety and Depression Association of America (ADAA), social anxiety disorder affects some 15 million Americans. In addition to social anxiety disorder, other types include generalized anxiety disorder, panic disorder, specific phobias, and separation anxiety disorder. Moreover, it is not unusual for people to experience more than one type of anxiety disorder.

Those who suffer from social anxiety disorder fear contact with others. In contrast, separation anxiety disorder afflicts people who are forced to leave the company of others whom they trust. The disorder affects mostly young children. A typical example may find a young child getting on the school bus for the first time, leaving the safety of home and his or her parents to go to school. The child may burst into tears and sob uncontrollably all the way to school—a reaction that could be interpreted as a panic attack. Most children grow out of the affliction once they become comfortable with their teachers and make new friends at school.

But sometimes separation anxiety does not go away. It continues to cling to a person, even into adulthood. And it can have harmful effects not only on the person suffering from separation anxiety but on that person's loved ones as well. Authors Vijaya Manicavasagar, a psychologist, and Derrick Silove, a psychiatrist, point out that "adults may suffer from severe and persistent fears of being separated from their loved ones as well, with their fears directed at their children, partners, parents or other close attachments. If these fears relate to their children, parents may become highly overprotective and unable to let them go off on their own."[20]

Moreover, young people may get used to the constant help and assistance their parents provide. When those parents are no longer close by, feelings of separation anxiety may surface in their children. Separation anxiety among college students who are away from their homes for the first time is very common. A study by Keene State College in New Hampshire surveyed three hundred college freshmen nationwide and found that many students who described their parents as overprotective exhibited symptoms of anxiety. Julie Lythcott-Haims, the former dean of freshmen at Stanford University in California, explains,

> When parents have tended to do the stuff of life for kids — the waking up, the transporting, the reminding about deadlines and obligations, the bill-paying, the question-asking, the decision-making, the responsibility-taking, the talking to strangers, and the confronting of authorities, kids may be in for quite a shock when parents turn them loose in the world of college or work. They will experience setbacks, which will feel to them like failure.[21]

A study published in 2020 by the National Institutes of Health reported that approximately 6.6 percent of American adults have experienced separation anxiety disorder at some point in their lives, meaning the disorder could affect about 13 million people.

Generalized Anxiety Disorder

Anxiety disorders go beyond occasions in which people fear interactions with others or separation from loved ones. In many cases, people may succumb to excessive anxiety or worry about issues such as their health, employment, schoolwork, and everyday routine life circumstances as well as interactions with others. This condition is known as generalized anxiety disorder.

People who suffer from generalized anxiety disorder may constantly feel restless, as if they are always wound up or on edge. They may tire easily and have difficulty concentrating. They may constantly feel irritable. Physical ailments may be present as well. People who suffer from generalized anxiety disorder may

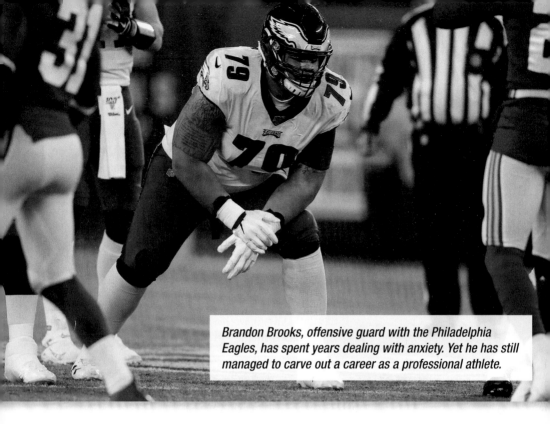

Brandon Brooks, offensive guard with the Philadelphia Eagles, has spent years dealing with anxiety. Yet he has still managed to carve out a career as a professional athlete.

feel muscle aches and have trouble sleeping. "You start to worry and grow noticeably apprehensive," write authors David Mellinger and Steven Jay Lynn. "Despite your efforts to shift your mood elsewhere, your uneasiness escalates. Before you know it, your mood has changed so that your anxious negativity seems to affect everything and everyone around you. Perhaps you also begin to experience your anxiety physically, tensing up and even undergoing some panic symptoms."[22] According to the ADAA, generalized anxiety disorder affects some 7 million Americans.

Panic Disorder

People who suffer from anxiety disorders may become so stressed that they feel overcome by their situations and experience dire physical symptoms. These symptoms include a pounding or racing heart, sweating, chills, trembling, difficulty breathing, weakness, dizziness, a tingling sensation or a numbness in their hands or fingers, chest pain, stomach pain, and nausea. These symptoms often manifest themselves if the person is going through a panic attack. If these attacks occur frequently, it is likely the person falls into the category of anxiety disorder known as panic disorder. According to the ADAA, panic disorder affects about 6 million Americans.

Panic disorder is the category in which professional football player Brandon Brooks has found himself. Brooks has spent years dealing with anxiety, yet he has still managed to carve out a career as a professional athlete. In November 2019, Brooks took the field with his team, the Philadelphia Eagles, in a home game against the Seattle Seahawks. But midway through the game, Brooks left the field and returned to the locker room. After the game, he disclosed that he was struck by a panic attack. He posted this explanation of what happened on his Twitter account:

I woke up, and did my typical routine of morning vomiting. It didn't go away like it normally does, but I figured it would calm down once I got to the stadium. It did, but I felt exhausted. The nausea and vomiting came back until I left the field, and tried everything I could to get back for my teammates but just wasn't able to do it.

Make no mistake I'm not ashamed or embarrassed by this nor what I go through daily. I've had this under control for a couple years, and had a setback yesterday. The only thing I'm upset about is that when my team needed me, I wasn't able to be out there with and for them.[23]

Panic attacks are usually preceded by a specific stressful event in a person's life that causes that person to be nervous and

As far back as the era of ancient Greece, some twenty-five hundred years ago, physicians were able to recognize the symptoms of anxiety disorders. The pioneering Greek physician Hippocrates, who lived from 460 to 375 BCE, was the first to regard anxiety as a form of mental illness, coining the term *hysteria* to describe the affliction. In 1621 a British researcher, Robert Burton, described the condition in his book *The Anatomy of Melancholia*, observing prolonged periods of unhappiness in some people who were occasionally stricken by what he called the "foul fiend of fear," which caused them to turn "red, pale, tremble, sweat, it makes sudden cold and heat come over the body [and] palpitation of the heart."

In 1926, Austrian psychoanalyst Sigmund Freud offered the modern definition of anxiety disorders. Freud found that in people who suffer from anxiety disorders, relatively minor feelings of discomfort tend to snowball, eventually consuming them and often making them incapable of functioning. Freud used the German term *angst* to describe the condition. *Angst* and the English term *anxiety* trace their roots to the Latin *angustia*, the modern translation of which is "anguish."

Quoted in George Makari, "In the Arcadian Woods," *Opinionator* (blog), *New York Times*, April 16, 2012. https://opinionator.blogs.nytimes.com.

fearful. In Brooks's case, it was the game against the Seahawks. Others may experience panic attacks if they are diagnosed with diseases. Or they may be facing breakups with their romantic partners. Or perhaps a business deal has gone sour or they made errors at work that they fear could mean their dismissal. Mellinger and Lynn explain that "an anxiety-sensitive individual who goes through a stressful major event or episode is likely to experience lingering, heightened anxiety and is at increased risk for erupting into panic."[24]

Moreover, an anxiety-ridden person who experiences a panic attack is likely to possess a mental trigger, meaning his or her brain will react in panic if it concludes that the situation warrants that reaction. This means that if a person experiences one panic attack, it is likely he or she will experience more such attacks. "Once an individual's 'triggering mechanism' is cocked," write Mellinger and Lynn, "he or she is likely to suffer attacks unless the problem is solved or the trigger is disarmed by means of treatment."[25]

Specific Phobias

The physical symptoms displayed by Brooks during the game against the Seahawks were in no small part prompted by fear. In Brooks's case, it was the fear of not performing up to the demands expected of a professional athlete. But fear can be associated with many specific causes. These causes are known as phobias, and they can cause anxiety in people who come into contact with them. According to the ADAA,

> High bridges, new places, or old elevators may make us a bit uneasy or even frightened. We might try to avoid things that make us uncomfortable, but most people generally manage to control their fears and carry out daily activities without incident.

> But people with specific phobias, or strong irrational fear reactions, work hard to avoid common places, situations, or objects even though they know there's no threat or danger. The fear may not make any sense, but they feel powerless to stop it.[26]

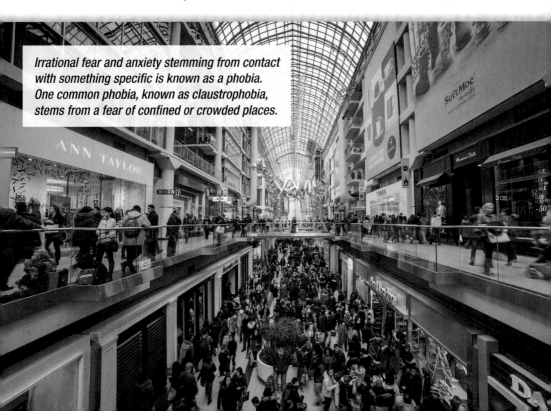

Irrational fear and anxiety stemming from contact with something specific is known as a phobia. One common phobia, known as claustrophobia, stems from a fear of confined or crowded places.

Among common phobias are claustrophobia (a fear of confined or crowded places), acrophobia (a fear of heights), and autophobia (a fear of being alone). Some less common phobias are arachnophobia (a fear of spiders), hydrophobia (a fear of water), and ophidiophobia (a fear of snakes).

Moreover, there is also a very general and all-encompassing phobia known as agoraphobia, which is commonly regarded as a fear of open places. But psychologists regard anyone with a fear of places or situations that triggers a sense of helplessness as suffering from agoraphobia. Essentially, a person who suffers from agoraphobia can be overcome by anxiety in virtually any situation that causes discomfort. It could happen while waiting in line at a supermarket, traveling on a train, or simply walking in a public park. Hal Mathew, a journalist from Salem, Oregon, who has suffered from agoraphobia for many years, says he suffered his first panic attack due to agoraphobia as a nineteen-year-old college student while on a road trip through rural Montana with several friends:

> We came out of a narrow canyon and emerged onto the land of never-ending openness—the Montana plains. They go on forever, flat and drab and suffocatingly frightening to a person like me. Those claiming normalcy would view the same wide-open spaces with probable boredom. Why the difference? We don't know, but the panic attack I had on the spot (and managed to conceal from my friends) was so scary that it prevented me from traveling freely again for another thirty years. . . . From that point on I felt a large black *A for agoraphobe* was branded onto my forehead.[27]

According to the ADAA, as many as 19 million Americans harbor phobias to some degree. And, certainly, most people are able to face their fears with little disruption to their daily lives. In the case of people who fear spiders, it is likely that most arachnophobes would simply walk away from the spiders they may see scurrying across the sidewalk rather than lapse into panic attacks. But still, as Mathew experienced, specific phobias can cause panic attacks. He says, "Once you have a couple of panic attacks and the indescribable fear they bring, you live in dread that you might have another, at any moment and with no warning. This keeps you on edge and, therefore, more likely to have another panic attack. It's a cruel, consuming cycle."[28]

In modern culture, fears seem to be everywhere. Whereas some people fear meeting new people, others fear separating from the people they love. Some people fear making mistakes at school that could cost them good grades. Even simple, everyday objects and experiences, such as spiders, elevator rides, and very small rooms, prompt feelings of anxiety in people. And when people find they can no longer contain those feelings, they succumb to physical ills such as racing heartbeats, vomiting, dizziness, and numbness in their hands and fingers—all symptoms of panic attacks. Certainly, many people are able to confront their fears and live normal lives, but for millions of others, anxiety disorders are daily burdens they must bear.

> "The panic attack I had on the spot (and managed to conceal from my friends) was so scary that it prevented me from traveling freely again for another thirty years."[27]
>
> —Hal Mathew, who suffers from agoraphobia

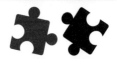

Chapter Three

What Causes Anxiety and Anxiety Disorders?

Tessa Miller suffered her first panic attack at the age of twenty-four. She was working on her laptop in her apartment in Brooklyn, New York. Suddenly, Miller felt the heavy beats of her heart. Her chest heaved as she found herself taking deep breaths. Her hands started trembling and her vision turned blurry. "Suddenly, I was hot and sweaty, so hot and sweaty that I stripped off my sweatshirt and went to run my face under cold water," she says.

> But as I stood up to go to the sink, the hand trembling traveled down into my arms and legs, leaving me unsteady on my feet. My heart seemed to pound even faster, even harder. I tried taking a deep breath to calm myself, but my breaths were sharp and shallow. My vision got darker and narrower and looked kaleidoscopic, like when you close your eyes and press down on your eyelids to "see stars."
>
> "You're dying," a voice in my head said. "This is what death feels like, and you're going to die alone."[29]

Three months before Miller suffered the panic attack, she had been hospitalized with severe abdominal pain. She was diagnosed then with Crohn's disease, an affliction that causes inflammation in a person's bowels. People who suffer from Crohn's disease may experience severe pain, diarrhea, fatigue, and weight loss.

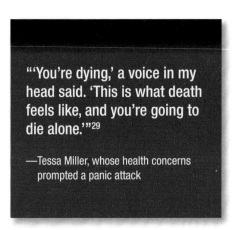

People with Crohn's disease can often manage their symptoms by watching their diets and taking prescription medications. Still, the symptoms can surface from time to time, meaning that at any time people with Crohn's disease can find themselves in pain and distress. Because of the pain and other physical ills that can surface at any time, people with Crohn's disease can lead stressful lives. And in Miller's case, that stress led to feelings of anxiety, which sparked the panic attack that suddenly afflicted her at what was otherwise a normal day at home performing some routine work on her laptop.

Miller believes the stress of worrying about the years ahead of her with Crohn's disease finally overwhelmed her, prompting her panic attack. Looking back on her life, Miller says many issues had caused her to feel anxious in years past, including a father who suffered from alcoholism, the divorce of her parents, and the deaths of family members. Miller says she had been carrying around an imaginary bucket for years, and all of those stressful experiences in her life were filling the bucket. After being diagnosed with Crohn's disease, Miller believes the bucket finally overflowed, resulting in the panic attack. "Everyone carries around these heavy buckets," she says. "One bucket might be a traumatic childhood, another an abusive relationship, a third the loss of a loved one, the fourth an unfulfilling career. Add to that mix incurable illness, a very full bucket that you must carry with you the rest of your life, and it becomes too unwieldly to carry alone."[30]

Somatic Symptom Disorder

As Miller's case illustrates, fears about a debilitating illness can grow into an anxiety disorder. People whose anxiety disorders are sparked by the fear of illness may pay close and even undue attention to what are otherwise normal bodily functions. They may constantly take their own temperatures or pulse rates and fret over minor aches and pains. If they wake up with headaches, they may interpret the symptom as indicative of much more serious illnesses, prompting frequent trips to their doctors' offices or even hospital emergency rooms.

Psychologists apply the term *somatic symptom disorder* to such cases. People who suffer from somatic symptom disorder may feel their anxiety build to the point of panic. As medical journalist Marie Miguel writes, "A person with somatic symptom disorder could experience a panic attack. Their chest hurts, and they feel

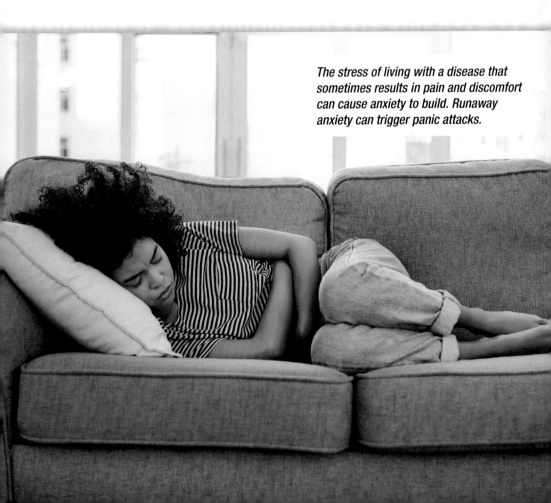

The stress of living with a disease that sometimes results in pain and discomfort can cause anxiety to build. Runaway anxiety can trigger panic attacks.

People who suffer from anxiety disorders often turn to alcohol and drugs to find solace from their anguish. According to the ADAA, 20 percent of people who suffer from anxiety disorders also develop addictions to alcohol and drugs.

But abusing alcohol and drugs can also cause feelings of anxiety. Many psychologists recognize a condition known as substance- or medication-induced anxiety as an anxiety disorder. When people become intoxicated through drinking or drug abuse, their thoughts can become scrambled. Under the influence of drugs and alcohol, minor feelings of anxiety can mushroom. People who abuse alcohol and drugs may find such episodes becoming a regular part of their lives. Psychologist Elizabeth Hartney explains,

> Unfortunately, the same drugs that many people use to try and boost their confidence, help them relax, and lower their inhibitions are the ones most prone to causing substance-induced anxiety disorder or panic attacks. In some cases, people don't even realize that it is alcohol, drugs, or medications that are causing anxiety because they only associate those substances with feeling good.

Elizabeth Hartney, "Substance/Medication-Induced Anxiety Disorder," Verywell Mind, November 20, 2020. www.verywellmind.com.

tightness in their stomach, and they are convinced that they [are having] a heart attack. In reality, they're having an anxiety attack."[31]

Although some people who suffer from anxiety fret over illnesses that are not real, there are certainly many people, among them Miller, whose illnesses are very real, causing them to feel anguish. When this anguish becomes a regular part of their lives, they may find themselves afflicted with generalized anxiety disorder.

The Pandemic Sparks Anxiety Attacks

Starting in early 2020, perhaps no disease created more anxiety among Americans and others than COVID-19. Caused by a deadly coronavirus, the disease spread throughout the world, becoming an international pandemic. Within a year of the outbreak of the disease in the city of Wuhan, China, more than 131 million people had been infected with the virus, including more than 2.8 million people who lost their lives to the disease. In America, by the spring of 2021 COVID-19 had infected nearly 32 million people and resulted in more than 570,000 deaths.

To help prevent the spread of the disease in America and elsewhere, government officials ordered lockdowns, closing many businesses, recreational venues, and other public places. People were forced to stay home for long periods, which, in many cases, caused boredom and feelings of being confined. And when they did go out, people were often required to wear masks to reduce the spread of germs as well as maintain social distancing rules—remaining 6 feet (1.8 m) away from one another. News coverage of the pandemic dominated the media, with many news outlets posting daily updates on the number of people infected as well as the number of fatalities.

All of this served to spark widespread feelings of anxiety among many people. Psychologists reported many individuals calling their practices, seeking help with their fears that they or family members would become infected. "It makes sense because, as a culture, we have never spent so much time reading, talking, watching or learning about a specific issue related to our physical health," says Kimberly Presley, a psychologist in Dallas, Texas. "And a feeling of helplessness or lack of control coupled with real fear is a perfect recipe for anxiety."[32]

> "A feeling of helplessness or lack of control coupled with real fear is a perfect recipe for anxiety."[32]
>
> —Kimberly Presley, psychologist

Evidence suggests that young people were hit hardest by feelings of anxiety during the COVID-19 pandemic. Across America, schools and universities closed their in-person classes. Although most schools provided virtual classes through internet connections, many students reported feelings of abandonment and stress. Moreover, young adults just starting their careers were among those most likely to lose their jobs during the pandemic because many employers elected to provide their few remaining jobs to workers with seniority. A 2021 study published by the Kaiser Family Foundation, which studies health-related issues, found that 56 percent of Americans between the ages of eighteen and twenty-four reported mental health issues, including anxiety, during the first year of the pandemic. According to the Kaiser Family Foundation study,

> There are a variety of ways the pandemic has likely affected mental health, particularly with widespread social isolation resulting from necessary safety measures. A broad body of research links social isolation and loneliness to both poor

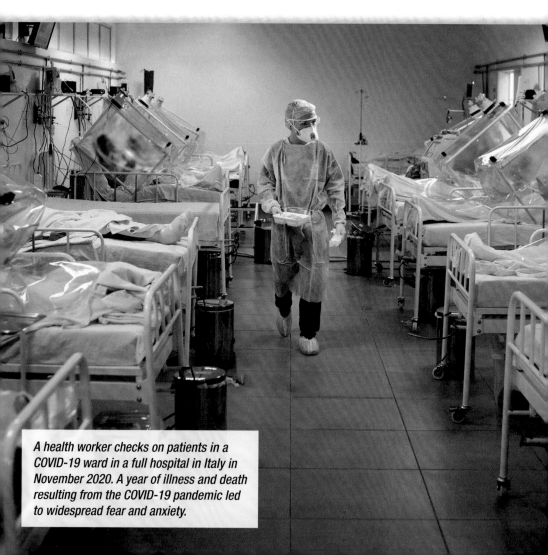

A health worker checks on patients in a COVID-19 ward in a full hospital in Italy in November 2020. A year of illness and death resulting from the COVID-19 pandemic led to widespread fear and anxiety.

mental and physical health. The widespread experience of loneliness became a public health concern even before the pandemic, given its association with reduced lifespan and greater risk of both mental and physical illnesses. . . .

Shortly after many stay-at-home orders were issued . . . those sheltering-in-place were more likely to report negative mental health effects resulting from worry or stress related to [COVID-19] compared to those not sheltering-in-place.[33]

Post-Traumatic Stress Disorder

Many people regarded the COVID-19 pandemic as a traumatic event in their lives. But even before the pandemic and, certainly, throughout the many months that COVID-19 dominated people's lives, other traumatic events could very well spark feelings of anxiety. In these cases, though, the traumatic events are specific to individuals. After the events have passed, these individuals continue to carry the burden of what they experienced. And that burden often manifests itself in feelings of anxiety.

When people harbor deeply intense and disturbing thoughts after a traumatic event in their lives, it is likely they are suffering from a condition known as post-traumatic stress disorder (PTSD). They may relive these events through flashbacks or nightmares. They may be overcome by feelings of sadness, fear, and anger. Ordinary events, such as a popping noise or accidental touch by another person, may serve as reminders of traumatic events, prompting PTSD sufferers to experience panic attacks. The condition is common among veterans who fought in battle in Afghanistan, Iraq, and other war zones. During their tours of duty, they were exposed to violence, bloodshed, and the loss of friends who died in battle. They may very well have taken the lives of enemy soldiers as part of their missions. Returning home, they remain troubled by all they witnessed on the battlefield, and many veterans find themselves suffering from PTSD. A 2015 US Department of Veterans Affairs study reported that 13.5 percent of military

Airplanes and Anxiety

Airplanes used in commercial flights are pressurized because they travel at heights of 33,000 feet (10,058 m) or more, where the atmosphere is thin. Thus, oxygen is pumped throughout the plane's cabin to enable people to breathe. Even though the cabin is pressurized, the air pressure is still a bit below what is common at sea level. In fact, the air pressure in an airplane cabin is typically similar to what a hiker may experience atop an 8,000-foot (2,348 m) mountain.

Most people hardly notice the difference, but in some people, the thinner atmosphere inside the cabin causes mild cases of hypoxia, or a lack of oxygen. Symptoms of hypoxia include headaches, shortness of breath, faster heartbeats, coughing, wheezing, and confusion. And when some people notice those symptoms, they may be prone to feelings of anxiety, resulting in a panic attack aboard the plane. Science journalist Maria Cohut explains that "research has demonstrated that high-altitude hypoxia, which is a slight decrease in oxygen supply, might naturally increase a sense of anxiety, so while you're in no danger whatsoever, you may feel unease as if you were under threat."

Maria Cohut, "How Can You Cope with Fear of Flying?," Medical News Today, December 14, 2017. www.medical newstoday.com.

members who served in Afghanistan and Iraq—about 350,000 veterans who served in the two wars dating back to 2001—have suffered from symptoms of PTSD.

But even people who have not been involved in military missions can suffer from PTSD. Eric, a thirteen-year-old in Canada, was diagnosed with PTSD. In Eric's case, the traumatic incident that led to his anxiety was a car crash. He was riding in a car driven by his mother when another driver ran a red light and smashed into their car. The collision forced their car to spin several times and smash into a tree. Miraculously, neither Eric nor his mother sustained injuries. However, the other driver was seriously injured. When Eric emerged from his mother's car, he could see blood covering the other driver's head and face. "[It was] like a color picture in my head,"[34] recalls Eric.

Because of the accident, Eric refuses to ride in cars. He is even terrified of walking on sidewalks next to streets. "[There are] crazy drivers everywhere,"[35] he says. When he does leave his home, he insists that his mother accompany him; when she is not with him, he suffers from separation anxiety disorder. In the year since the accident, Eric has dropped out of karate class and quit his soccer team—two activities he thoroughly enjoyed—because going to those activities would require him to ride in a car. Moreover, Eric suffers from frequent nightmares and has experienced panic attacks when he hears the sound of a car horn. He will not even watch television out of fear that a news story about a car accident will be aired.

Chemical Imbalances

Serious illness and trauma are viewed as triggering events for anxiety and anxiety disorders. But many people who have these and other similar experiences develop levels of anxiety that they eventually overcome. Why, then, do some people become consumed by their anxieties? Mental health experts suggest that a chemical imbalance in the brain might make some individuals more likely to develop uncontrollable anxiety.

The human brain contains millions of cells that are known as neurons. Each neuron emits an electrical impulse that carries the brain's message, perhaps instructing the foot to take a step, the lips to form words, or the fingers to grasp a baseball. Carrying the electrical impulses from neuron to neuron are chemicals in the brain known as neurotransmitters.

Neurotransmitters do more than help the brain send signals to fingers, feet, and lips. They also control emotions. The neurotransmitter dopamine is known to regulate mood. Another neurotransmitter, serotonin, is known to affect levels of anger and aggression. Serotonin is also believed to be very involved in the brain's fight-or-flight response.

Research has suggested that people who suffer from excessive anxiety may have some sort of chemical imbalance in the brain. They may have too much, or too little, of the chemicals that control emotions, such as dopamine and serotonin. Mental health experts are quick to add, however, that the research is hardly definitive.

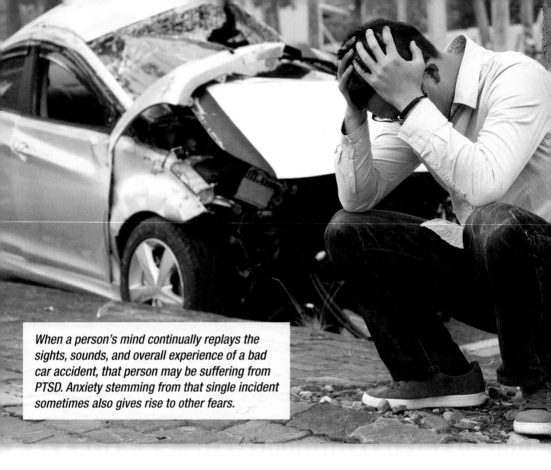

When a person's mind continually replays the sights, sounds, and overall experience of a bad car accident, that person may be suffering from PTSD. Anxiety stemming from that single incident sometimes also gives rise to other fears.

Many people who suffer from anxiety are not afflicted with neurotransmitter imbalances. Moreover, some experts also point out that repeated anxiety attacks may actually be causing neurotransmitter imbalances. According to psychologist Micah Abraham,

> It gets complicated. It does seem that many people seem to have risk factors for naturally low serotonin levels, and it's likely that many people are born with low serotonin, indicating that they are at a higher risk of developing anxiety. It's not just serotonin either—most neurotransmitters influence anxiety in some way, and in some cases an overabundance of a chemical can lead to anxiety.

> If you have anxiety you can also develop chemical imbalances that were not previously present, because anxiety

affects your brain chemicals. The way you think about your feelings and situations in your life is known, without a doubt, to influence whether problematic releases of serotonin . . . and other brain chemicals occur. It is possible to develop anxiety first, resulting in chemical imbalances.[36]

Is Anxiety Inherited?

Like other physical traits, such as eye color, hair color, physique, and even the shape of one's nose, it is likely that children inherit the levels of neurotransmitters in their brains from their parents. Therefore, many mental health experts have suggested that anxiety, like the color of one's eyes, may be an inherited trait. If a mother or father suffered from anxiety, chances are enhanced that a son or daughter would also be afflicted by uncontrollable fears and anguish.

A 2019 study published in the journal *Molecular Psychiatry* found that in 26 percent of cases studied by researchers, people who experienced recurrent bouts of anxiety had parents who also experienced high levels of anxiety. However, researchers are not yet certain whether anxiety is a product of one's genes—the chemical units in the body that provide the code for physical and mental characteristics—or the product of one's environment while growing up. In other words, if a young child grows up in an environment where a parent constantly endures anxiety attacks, that young child may very well come to react to

> "It might be genes or it may be because a family member modeled a very anxious way of being in the world—or often a combination of both."[37]
>
> —Elena Touroni, psychologist

stressful situations in the same way. "Family provides both the genes and the environment," says psychologist Elena Touroni. "It might be genes or it may be because a family member modeled a very anxious way of being in the world—or often a combination of both. It can be difficult to disentangle genes and environment."[37]

41

Research suggests that people experience anxiety due to several factors. Perhaps they have inherited their anxiety from their parents, either through chemical imbalances that were passed on genetically or because of the anxious environment in which they were raised. For others, it might have been traumatic events that sparked their anxiety, such as witnessing carnage on the battlefield, surviving a serious automobile accident, or realizing that that they will be living with a debilitating disease for the rest of their lives. And for many people, their anxiety grew out of the realization that they were imprisoned in a society afflicted by a pandemic that took the lives of millions of people—certainly a once-in-a-lifetime traumatic event that caused widespread anxiety throughout the world.

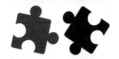

Chapter Four

Keeping Anxiety Under Control

Jenny Beck endured some difficult years in high school and college as she studied for a career as a physician. Whenever the date for an exam approached, Beck found herself growing anxious. "I feel the anxiety in the pit of my stomach," she says. "A bowling ball of stress, weighing me down and squeezing my insides. My heart pounds. My breathing is shallow. My body is in full 'flight or fight' mode, my [brain] priming me to fight for my survival. Am I about to plunge over a waterfall, escape an attacker or fight off a snake? No, I am about to take a test."[38]

Beck suffered from test anxiety. Although not ranked as an anxiety disorder, test anxiety afflicts many students. No matter how hard they study or how thoroughly they prepare for the test, they still lapse into fret-filled states as the dates of their exams draw near.

There are several reasons students experience test anxiety. They might not feel they have fully prepared for the test. Or they may be doing poorly in the class and, despite working hard to catch up, still fret that the coming test will result in another poor grade. Finally, students who suffer from test anxiety may harbor general fears of failure that manifest themselves in many corners of their lives, not just the classroom. In such cases, an approaching test is simply another reason for the student to feel anxious.

Despite how well students may have studied and prepared for the coming exams, test anxiety often robs them of the ability to concentrate. This begins an unfortunate cycle: unable to focus on the test questions, students do poorly on the exam, which then leads to a poor grade, which then heightens their feelings of anxiety—and sometimes becomes a full-blown panic attack.

Overcoming Test Anxiety

Despite enduring years of test anxiety, Beck was able to complete high school and college and launch her career as a physician. She was able to excel in her studies because she finally figured out ways to quell her test anxiety. Among her strategies was to resist cramming for tests—to pull the so-called all-nighters in which students stay up until the early morning hours before a test, studying hard. After an all-nighter, students are likely to walk into the classroom having slept little the night before, which is hardly a recipe for success when one is faced with a challenging exam. Instead, Beck says she found herself much more prepared for her tests by consistently working hard to learn the material as it was presented by her teachers. In fact, Beck says, she found herself better prepared for the tests if she got a good night's sleep beforehand rather than spending those late-night hours cramming for her exams.

> "I feel the anxiety in the pit of my stomach. A bowling ball of stress, weighing me down and squeezing my insides."[38]
>
> —Jenny Beck, a physician who overcame her test anxiety

She pursued other commonsense strategies as well. She made sure she ate a good meal before a test because she found that hunger often distracted her, and distractions often fed her anxieties. She took deep breaths as she sat down to take the tests in class. Physicians know that deep breathing aids in concentration because it activates what is known as the parasympathetic nervous system in the body. The parasympathetic nervous system is sparked by brain cells that control relaxation;

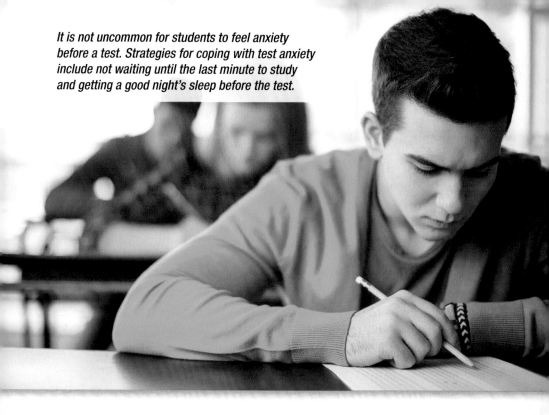

It is not uncommon for students to feel anxiety before a test. Strategies for coping with test anxiety include not waiting until the last minute to study and getting a good night's sleep before the test.

therefore, deep breathing helps many people relax. In contrast, taking shallow breaths, which anxious people tend to do, particularly during a panic attack, helps push people into the fight-or-flight mode. Once in flight mode, students are unlikely to be able to focus on the test.

Those strategies, plus keeping a positive attitude, worked for Beck. She says,

> Tell yourself that you studied hard and you know the information. Picture yourself leaving the testing area feeling happy and confident. What we believe becomes our reality. Try to only allow for positive thoughts. And keep things in perspective. A failed exam doesn't mean a failed life. It is only a chance to do better the next time. Keep a positive mindset and believe that you will do well on your exam but know that a missed question or a poor result is not the end of the world. Persistence often produces greater results than talent.[39]

Strategies for Easing Anxiety

People may find that some of those strategies—getting a good night's sleep, eating well, and taking deep breaths—work for forms of anxiety other than test anxiety. According to the ADAA, other common strategies include taking a time-out—in other words, take a step back from a situation that might be causing anxiety. And during that time-out, find relaxing things to do, such as listening to music, reading, gardening, or taking a walk.

Consuming alcoholic beverages can fuel anxious feelings because alcohol can change the neurotransmitter levels in the brain that control moods. Therefore, to avoid anxiety, people would do well to stay away from wine, liquor, and beer. Caffeine—the key ingredient in coffee—can also affect the chemical balance of neurotransmitters. Therefore, mental health experts counsel anxious people to cut down on or eliminate drinking coffee.

Cognitive Behavioral Therapy for Specific Phobias

People who suffer from specific phobias, such as claustrophobia (a fear of confined places) or acrophobia (a fear of heights), may be advised by psychologists to undergo cognitive behavioral therapy (CBT). In simple terms, CBT requires someone with a specific fear to take gradual steps toward conquering that fear. For example, patients with acrophobia may be advised to gradually work their way up flights of steps until they feel new levels of comfort as they climb higher. Finally, they may find themselves standing comfortably on the outdoor deck of a tall building with no feelings of anxiety. As psychologist Ellen Bowers explains,

> If a person is terrified of flying he might first look at pictures of airplanes, and then watch films of planes. Next, he might book a flight with a helpful, supportive companion, friend, or therapist. It could be a short jaunt to a nearby city. The person might . . . mentally rehearse each part of the experience—checking in, checking the luggage, going through security, waiting near the gate, boarding the plane. . . . This mental rehearsal conditions the mind and body to be calm and unsurprised with each step of the process. The final step is to take the actual flight.

Ellen Bowers, *The Everything Guide to Cognitive Behavioral Therapy*. New York: Adams Media, 2013, p. 56.

Exercise offers another way of managing anxiety. Since anxiety is often driven by concerns about health, it makes sense that healthy people may be less anxious. And a way to stay healthy is to get plenty of exercise. Moreover, mental health experts agree that when people are fully engaged in exercise, they tend to focus on their workouts, which means they are not conjuring up anxious thoughts. Exercise, therefore, can offer a healthy distraction from troubling thoughts.

Learning to laugh is another strategy for coping with anxiety. According to the ADAA, a good sense of humor goes a long way toward controlling feelings of anxiety.

Keeping a journal, the ADAA notes, can also help people manage anxiety. Many times, people who suffer from anxiety do not know what triggers anxious feelings. A journal offers a place to take note of events that spark those feelings. Once the triggering events become clear, individuals can develop their own personal strategies for avoiding those situations or confronting them with positive attitudes.

Confiding in friends can also be helpful. Very often, anxious people keep their fears bottled up inside. Mental health experts believe anxious people can find a measure of relief by stating their worries out loud to someone they trust. Good friends will often provide needed words of encouragement.

A final strategy for managing anxiety, the ADAA states, is to face reality. It is important to realize that no one can control all of the events in his or her life. The ADAA says to "do your best. Instead of aiming for perfection, which isn't possible, be proud of however close you get. Accept that you cannot control everything. Put your stress in perspective: Is it really as bad as you think?"[40]

Coping with Anxiety Disorders

Although those strategies may help people deal with their everyday anxieties, people who suffer from deeper feelings of worry and fear—those classified as anxiety disorders—may have to take further steps to confront their troubles. They may need to seek help from psychologists or other mental health professionals. Since many anxious people do not know what is sparking their fret-filled feelings, they may require the expertise of psychologists to get to the root of their problems and offer coping strategies. Psychologist Suzanne Gelb describes what occurs during a typical session with an anxiety patient:

> Each session is, essentially, a problem-solving session. You describe your current situation, and your feelings about it, and then the therapist uses their expertise to assist you in trying to resolve that problem so you can move closer to having the life you wish to have.
>
> At the beginning of a session, the therapist typically invites you to share what's been going on in your life, what's on your mind, what's bothering you, or whether there are any

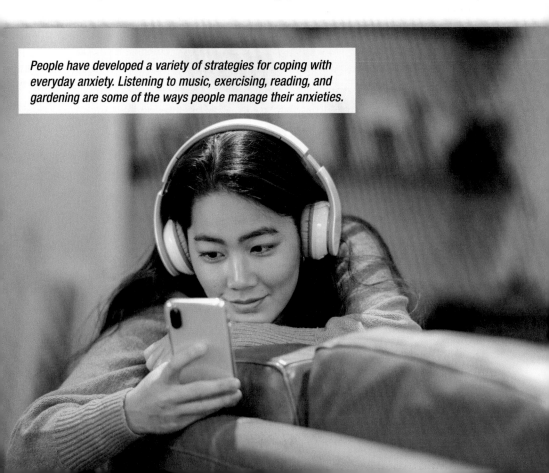

People have developed a variety of strategies for coping with everyday anxiety. Listening to music, exercising, reading, and gardening are some of the ways people manage their anxieties.

goals you'd like to discuss. You'll be invited to speak openly. The therapist will listen and may take notes as you speak; some, like myself, take notes after a session. You won't be criticized, interrupted or judged as you speak. Your conversation will be kept in the strictest confidentiality. This is a special, unique type of conversation in which you can say exactly what you feel—total honesty—without worrying that you're going to hurt someone's feelings, damage a relationship, or be penalized in any way. Anything you want—or need—to say is OK.[41]

Anxiety Medications

Counseling helps many people suffering from anxiety disorders, but overcoming an anxiety disorder often also requires medication. In people who have anxiety disorders, medication can help solve neurotransmitter imbalances. The two most common antianxiety drugs are known as selective serotonin reuptake inhibitors (SSRIs) and benzodiazepines.

As the name suggests, SSRI drugs work by controlling the amount of serotonin in the brain. Specifically, SSRI drugs block brain cells from absorbing serotonin, meaning high levels of serotonin remain in the patient's nervous system. Because high levels of serotonin can help ease tensions, SSRI drugs can be effective in controlling anxiety. The drug Zoloft is one of the most common SSRI medications that is prescribed by physicians.

"This is a special, unique type of conversation in which you can say exactly what you feel—total honesty—without worrying that you're going to hurt someone's feelings, damage a relationship, or be penalized in any way."[41]

—Suzanne Gelb, psychologist

Benzodiazepines are tranquilizers, meaning they promote relaxation. Specifically, they enhance the flow of the neurotransmitter gamma-aminobutyric acid, which tends to slow down messages carried from brain cell to brain cell. When these messages

49

are slowed down, they promote feelings of relaxation and, therefore, fewer feelings of anxiety. The most common benzodiazepine drugs that physicians prescribe are Valium and Xanax.

Courtenay Hameister, the former radio host who suffered her first moment of anxiety on a public pool diving board at the age of eight, believes the pressures of her broadcasting job caused her to develop generalized anxiety disorder. For twelve years she hosted *Live Wire!*, a weekly radio show taped on Saturdays in front of an audience and broadcast on the National Public Radio network. Before stepping down in 2015, Hameister's duties called on her to interview newsmakers—many of whom were prize-winning authors, filmmakers, and other celebrities. As the taping day for the show approached, Hameister could feel the anxiety build up inside her as she feared she would fail to ask the right questions, be entertaining, amuse the audience, and otherwise host a successful episode of the show.

> "This wasn't a mild anxiety attack, though. I was still the aforementioned ball of electrified wires, but the Xanax helped to keep the voltage below two hundred."[42]
>
> —Courtenay Hameister, who took Xanax to cope with her anxiety

Finally, her physician prescribed Xanax. Hameister took her first dose as she felt herself consumed by a panic attack. "When you're having a mild anxiety attack, [Xanax is] like perspective in a pill," she says. "Once you've taken it, all the thoughts that used to be racing are now sitting quietly drinking tea. . . . This wasn't a mild anxiety attack, though. I was still the aforementioned ball of electrified wires, but the Xanax helped to keep the voltage below two hundred."[42]

Addictions to Antianxiety Drugs

Although medication can go a long way toward chemically controlling the neurotransmitter imbalances that may be at the root of anxiety disorders, a downside to prescription drugs is that they can be addictive. Indeed, with so many millions of people suf-

Brain Surgery for OCD

For more than twenty years, some victims of the debilitating brain disorder Parkinson's disease have found relief in a procedure known as deep brain stimulation. To perform the procedure, physicians surgically implant a device known as an electrode into the brain. The electronic pulses emitted by the device can be effective in controlling the symptoms of Parkinson's disease, including shaking, stiffness, and difficulty with walking, balance, and coordination.

In recent years, some patients afflicted with severe cases of OCD have also been treated with surgically implanted electrodes. The pulses emitted by the device are found to be effective in controlling mood and, therefore, the feelings of anxiety experienced by OCD patients. At the University of Colorado Hospital in Aurora, Colorado, a patient named Jon underwent the procedure after suffering for years from OCD. Finding himself harboring anxieties about cleanliness, he obsessively washed his hands. After receiving the implant, Jon was able to pursue a normal life. Whenever he senses symptoms of OCD approaching, Jon activates the electrode and soon finds his symptoms easing. "Just the feeling of pushing a button and have your brain feel like it's climbing—I wish other people could experience it," he says.

Quoted in Todd Neff, "Deep Brain Stimulation Zaps OCD, Opens New Path for Young Patient," UCHealth, December 19, 2019. www.uchealth.org.

fering from anxiety disorders, physicians are writing millions of prescriptions a year for people who need drugs to help control their symptoms. And many of those patients may find themselves addicted to those drugs.

Benzodiazepine drugs can be addictive because they tend to become less effective the more they are used. This means that many patients may have to take more frequent and larger doses of benzodiazepines to continue to control their anxiety disorder symptoms. In most cases, benzodiazepine drugs are not taken daily; patients are instructed to take the drugs only when they begin experiencing their symptoms of anxiety. But as they take more frequent and larger doses of the pills, it is very likely that patients may find themselves taking their benzodiazepine drugs every day, or even more than once per day.

SSRI drugs are not considered to be addictive, but they have their downsides as well. Unlike benzodiazepine drugs, physicians prescribe SSRI drugs to be taken once daily. (Some patients may

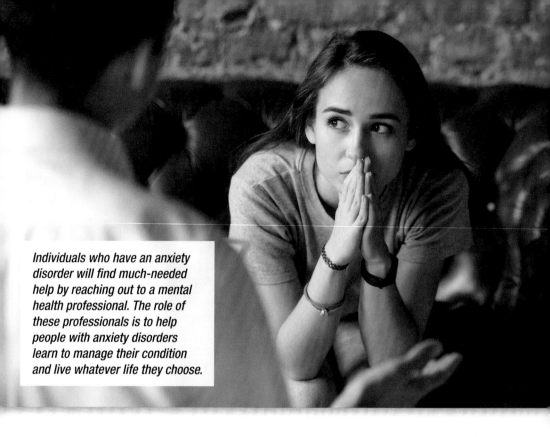

Individuals who have an anxiety disorder will find much-needed help by reaching out to a mental health professional. The role of these professionals is to help people with anxiety disorders learn to manage their condition and live whatever life they choose.

be instructed to take more than one dose per day.) Usually, patients will spend several months on their SSRI prescriptions. When physicians believe their patients' anxiety disorders are under control, they may reduce or eliminate the prescriptions. Although doctors may try to gradually reduce the dosages, sometimes patients still experience physical and emotional effects of drug withdrawal. This can include headaches, restlessness, insomnia, fatigue, irritability, and, perhaps, a relapse of anxiety disorder symptoms.

Fears of Illness

Hameister believes her generalized anxiety disorder was prompted by fears of illness—specifically, dementia. Common mostly in elderly people, dementia is a decline in cognitive abilities. Among the symptoms of dementia is forgetfulness. Sometimes, people's memories can be so blocked by dementia that they lose the ability to function, forgetting to eat, getting lost in their own neighborhoods, and failing to recognize their own family members. In Hameister's case, her anxiety about dementia occurred shortly after she turned forty. This is decades before she would have typically experienced the symptoms of dementia if, in fact, she ever developed those symptoms. Hameister attributes her fear of approaching dementia to occasional, brief lapses of memory, which are common among people of all ages. However, she came to believe those minor lapses in memory were symptoms of dementia.

Finally, she underwent a brain scan that showed no signs that her mental functions were deteriorating. Greatly relieved, Hameister decided to confront her anxieties rather than continuing to depend on medication. She realized that she had been taking larger and more frequent doses to control the symptoms and that this actually might be contributing to her anxieties. So she decided to give up her Xanax prescription. "When I went off the Xanax, I stopped worrying that I had a degenerative brain disease," she says.

> But I learned something. . . . I learned that when you have [anxiety], even if you're not feeling anxious, your anxiety is free-floating, just hanging around waiting for something to attach to. I knew that from now on, I needed to manage my anxiety or it would blossom into . . . episodes whenever I went through a big life change like moving, getting a new job, or a death in the family. Not exactly ideal times to have massive, crippling anxiety.[43]

Anxiety is a normal human emotion. People experience it for different reasons and with varying levels of intensity. Whether people experience everyday anxiety or debilitating anxiety, it can be managed. Exercise, meditation, healthy diet, and other tools such as these have been shown to help people manage everyday anxiety. When anxiety escalates to the point of disrupting daily life, other tools are needed. These include mental health counseling and sometimes medication. These tools allow people to develop new perspectives and new routines so that anxiety does not take over their lives.

Source Notes

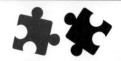

Introduction: Even Superheroes Suffer from Anxiety

1. Peter Travers, "*Deadpool*: Ryan Reynolds Brings Back His 'Merc with a Mouth' Superhero for Maximum (and Meta) Chaos," *Rolling Stone*, February 11, 2016. www.rollingstone.com.
2. Quoted in Cara Buckley, "This Story Has Already Stressed Ryan Reynolds Out," *New York Times*, May 2, 2018. www.nytimes.com.
3. Quoted in Buckley, "This Story Has Already Stressed Ryan Reynolds Out."
4. Quoted in ScienceDaily, "Even a Single Mindfulness Meditation Session Can Reduce Anxiety," April 23, 2018. www.sciencedaily.com.
5. Quoted in Buckley, "This Story Has Already Stressed Ryan Reynolds Out."

Chapter One: What Is Everyday Anxiety?

6. Scott Muska, "Real Guys Describe the Anxiety of Waiting for Girls to Text Them Back," *Women's Health*, October 2, 2015. www.womenshealthmag.com.
7. Lucie Hemmen, *The Teen Girl's Anxiety Survival Guide*: *Ten Ways to Conquer Anxiety and Feel Your Best*. Oakland, CA: New Harbinger, 2021, p. 6.
8. Zee Krstic, "How to Help Someone Struggling with Anxiety," *Good Housekeeping*, April 23, 2020. www.goodhousekeeping.com.
9. David Mellinger and Steven Jay Lynn, *The Monster in the Cave: How to Face Your Fear and Anxiety and Live Your Life*. New York: Berkley, 2003, p. 5.
10. Mellinger and Lynn, *The Monster in the Cave*, p. 50.
11. Courtenay Hameister, *Okay Fine Whatever: The Year I Went from Being Afraid of Everything to Only Being Afraid of Most Things*. New York: Little, Brown, 2018, p. 4.
12. Katie Hurley, "6 Hidden Signs of Teen Anxiety," Psycom, February 25, 2021. www.psycom.net.

13. Lisa Damour, *Under Pressure: Confronting the Epidemic of Stress and Anxiety in Girls*. New York: Ballantine, 2019, p. xvii.
14. Quoted in Damour, *Under Pressure*, p. 15.

Chapter Two: What Happens When Anxiety Becomes a Disorder?
15. Quoted in Barbara G. Markway and Gregory P. Markway, *Painfully Shy: How to Overcome Social Anxiety and Reclaim Your Life*. New York: Thomas Dunne, 2003, p. 12.
16. Quoted in Markway and Markway, *Painfully Shy*, p. 11.
17. Quoted in Markway and Markway, *Painfully Shy*, p. 11.
18. American Addiction Centers, "Pathological, Abnormal Anxiety." www.mentalhelp.net.
19. Quoted in Jenna Birch, "This Is the Difference Between Normal Anxiety and an Anxiety Disorder," HuffPost, November 13, 2020. www.huffpost.com.
20. Vijaya Manicavasagar and Derrick Silove, *Separation Anxiety Disorder in Adults: Clinical Features, Diagnostic Dilemmas and Treatment Guidelines*. London: Elsevier, 2020, p. xi.
21. Julie Lythcott-Haims, "Kids of Helicopter Parents Are Sputtering Out," *Slate*, July 5, 2015. https://slate.com.
22. Mellinger and Lynn, *The Monster in the Cave*, p. 204.
23. Quoted in Tyler Conway, "Eagles' Brandon Brooks Explains Anxiety Kept Him from Playing vs. Seahawks," BleacherReport, November 25, 2019. www.bleacherreport.com.
24. Mellinger and Lynn, *The Monster in the Cave*, p. 69.
25. Mellinger and Lynn, *The Monster in the Cave*, p. 69.
26. Anxiety and Depression Association of America, "Specific Phobias." https://adaa.org.
27. Hal Mathew, *Un-Agoraphobic: Overcome Anxiety, Panic Attacks, and Agoraphobia for Good*. San Francisco: Weiser, 2014, p. xxi.
28. Mathew, *Un-Agoraphobic*, p. ix.

Chapter Three: What Causes Anxiety and Anxiety Disorders?
29. Tessa Miller, "9 People Describe What It Feels Like to Have a Panic Attack," *Self*, October 28, 2017. www.self.com.
30. Tessa Miller, *What Doesn't Kill You: A Life with Chronic Illness—Lessons from a Body in Revolt*. New York: Henry Holt, 2021, pp. 98–99.
31. Marie Miguel, "Somatic Symptom Disorder Confuses Physical Symptoms with Danger," Good Men Project, January 20, 2021. https://goodmenproject.com.

32. Quoted in Nicole Pajer, "11 Sneaky Signs You Have Health Anxiety Because of the COVID-19 Pandemic," HuffPost, March 29, 2021. www.huffpost.com.
33. Nirmita Panchal et al., "The Implications of COVID-19 for Mental Health and Substance Use," Kaiser Family Foundation, February 10, 2021. www.kff.org.
34. Quoted in Anxiety Canada, "Eric's Story (PTSD)." www.anxiety canada.com.
35. Quoted in Anxiety Canada, "Eric's Story (PTSD)."
36. Micah Abraham, "Are Anxiety Disorders Caused by a Chemical Imbalance?," CalmClinic, October 10, 2020. www.calmclinic.com.
37. Quoted in Kelly Burch, "Is Anxiety Genetic? Anxiety Disorders Are Caused by a Combination of Both Genes and Your Environment," Insider, April 21, 2020. www.insider.com.

Chapter Four: Keeping Anxiety Under Control

38. Jenny Beck, "Study Better and Defeat Test Anxiety," Medium, August 13, 2019. https://medium.com.
39. Beck, "Study Better and Defeat Test Anxiety."
40. Anxiety and Depression Association of America, "Tips to Manage Anxiety and Stress." https://adaa.org.
41. Suzanne Gelb, "What Really Happens in a Therapy Session," *All Grown Up* (blog), *Psychology Today*, December 5, 2015. www .psychologytoday.com.
42. Hameister, *Okay Fine Whatever*, p. 271.
43. Hameister, *Okay Fine Whatever*, p. 276.

Anxiety and Depression Association of America (ADAA)

https://adaa.org

The ADAA provides many resources for people experiencing anxiety as well as students who are studying the causes of anxiety. By accessing the "For the Public" link, visitors can find articles defining the different anxiety disorders, among them generalized anxiety disorder, social anxiety disorder, panic disorder, and others.

Center for the Treatment and Study of Anxiety (CTSA)

www.med.upenn.edu/ctsa

A department of the University of Pennsylvania School of Medicine in Philadelphia, the CTSA's website provides many resources on anxiety, including articles on how to recognize symptoms of various anxiety disorders as well as an overview of the training involved for students who may be considering pursuing careers in psychology and the treatment of anxiety disorders.

Lisa Damour, PhD

www.drlisadamour.com

Psychologist Lisa Damour specializes in treating anxiety in teen girls and lists many resources about anxiety on her website. By accessing the "Articles" link, visitors can find dozens of news articles she has written on the topic that have appeared in publications such as *Your Teen Magazine*, the *New York Times*, and *Time* magazine.

National Institute of Mental Health (NIMH)

www.nimh.nih.gov

The NIMH is a federal agency that sponsors research into mental health issues, including anxiety. By entering the term "anxiety" into the website's search engine, visitors can find numerous articles about anxiety, including a 2021 study that identified risk factors that could spark anxieties in young people.

WorryWiseKids

www.worrywisekids.org

Sponsored by the Children's Center for Obsessive and Compulsive Disorder and Anxiety in Pennsylvania, this website offers many resources for young children and teens to help them deal with their anxiety issues. By accessing the link for "Anxiety 101," visitors can read about how everyday anxieties can evolve into anxiety disorders.

For Further Research

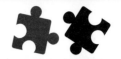

Books

Lisa Damour, *Under Pressure: Confronting the Epidemic of Stress and Anxiety in Girls*. New York: Ballantine, 2019.

Courtenay Hameister, *Okay Fine Whatever: The Year I Went from Being Afraid of Everything to Only Being Afraid of Most Things*. New York: Little, Brown, 2018.

Lucie Hemmen, *The Teen Girl's Anxiety Survival Guide: Ten Ways to Conquer Anxiety and Feel Your Best*. Oakland, CA: New Harbinger, 2021.

Eva Holland, *Nerve: Adventures in the Science of Fear*. New York: The Experiment, 2020.

Celina McManus, *Understanding Anxiety*. San Diego: ReferencePoint, 2020.

Internet Sources

Jenna Birch, "This Is the Difference Between Normal Anxiety and an Anxiety Disorder," HuffPost, November 13, 2020. www.huffpost.com.

Cara Buckley, "This Story Has Already Stressed Ryan Reynolds Out," *New York Times*, May 2, 2018. www.nytimes.com.

Katie Hurley, "6 Hidden Signs of Teen Anxiety," Psycom, February 25, 2021. www.psycom.net.

Tessa Miller, "9 People Describe What It Feels Like to Have a Panic Attack," *Self*, October 28, 2017. www.self.com.

Nicole Pajer, "11 Sneaky Signs You Have Health Anxiety Because of the COVID-19 Pandemic," HuffPost, March 29, 2021. www.huffpost.com.

Index

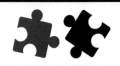

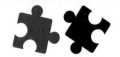

Hal Marcovitz is a former newspaper reporter and columnist who lives in Chalfont, Pennsylvania. He has written more than two hundred books for young readers.